C000048317

The Easy Plant-Based Guide to Tasty Sauces and Drinks

The Complete Plant-Based Recipe Book for Homemade Sauces and Drinks

Ben Goleman

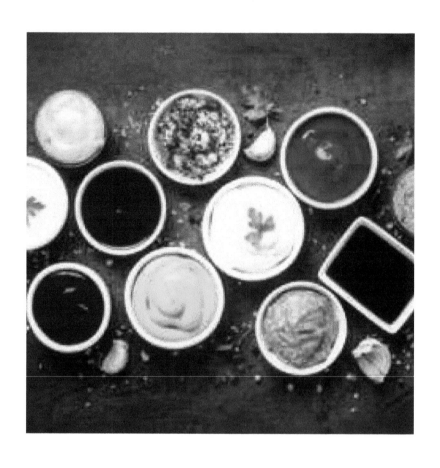

© Copyright 2021 - All rights reserved.

The content contained within this book may not be reproduced, duplicated or transmitted without direct written permission from the author or the publisher.

Under no circumstances will any blame or legal responsibility be held against the publisher, or author, for any damages, reparation, or monetary loss due to the information contained within this book. Either directly or indirectly.

Legal Notice:

This book is copyright protected. This book is only for personal use. You cannot amend, distribute, sell, use, quote or paraphrase any part, or the content within this book, without the consent of the author or publisher.

Disclaimer Notice:

Please note the information contained within this document is for educational and entertainment purposes only. All effort has been executed to present accurate, up to date, and reliable, complete information. No warranties of any kind are declared or implied. Readers acknowledge that the author is not engaging in the rendering of legal, financial, medical or professional dvice. The content within this book has been derived rom various sources. Please consult a licensed rofessional before attempting any techniques outlined in his book.

By reading this document, the reader agrees that under no circumstances is the author responsible for any losses, direct or indirect, which are incurred as a result of the use of information contained within this document, including, but not limited to, — errors, omissions, or inaccuracies.

Table of Contents

Coconut Peanut Butter Fudge

Servings: 20

Cooking Time: 0 Minute

Ingredients:

- 12 oz smooth peanut butter
- 3 tbsp coconut oil
- 4 tbsp coconut cream
- 15 drops liquid stevia
- Pinch of salt

Directions:

1. Line baking tray with parchment paper.
2. Melt coconut oil in a saucepan over low heat.
3. Add peanut butter, coconut cream, stevia, and salt in a saucepan. Stir well.
4. Pour fudge mixture into the prepared baking tray and place in refrigerator for 1 hour.
5. Cut into pieces and serve.

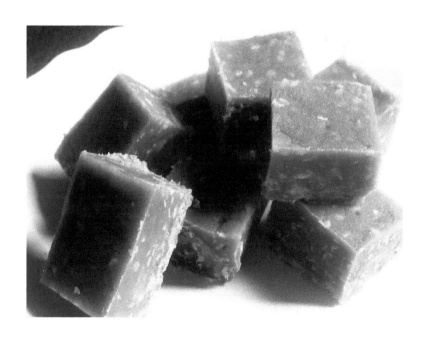

Kale And Walnut Pesto

Servings: 4

Cooking Time: 10 Minutes

Ingredients:

- 1/2 bunch kale, leaves chop
- 1/2 cup chopped walnuts
- 2 cloves of garlic, peeled
- 1/4 cup nutritional yeast
- ½ of lemon, juiced
- 1/4 cup olive oil
- ¼ teaspoon. ground black pepper
- 1/3 teaspoon. Salt

Directions:

1. Place a large pot filled with water over medium heat, bring it to boil, then add kale and boil for 5 minutes until tender.

2. Drain kale, then transfer it in a blender, add remaining ingredients and then pulse for 5 minutes until smooth.

3. Serve straight away.

Nutrition Info: Calories: 344 Cal; Fat: 29 g: Carbs: 16 g; Protein: 9 g; Fiber: 6 g

Thai-style Coconut Sauce

Servings: 4

Cooking Time: 10 Minutes

Ingredients:

*   1 tablespoon coconut oil
*   1 teaspoon garlic, minced
*   1 teaspoon fresh ginger, minced
*   1 lemon, juiced and zested
*   1 teaspoon turmeric powder
*   1/2 cup coconut milk
*   1 tablespoon soy sauce
*   1 teaspoon coconut sugar, or more to taste
*   A pinch of salt
*   A pinch of grated nutmeg

Directions:

1. In a small saucepan, melt the coconut oil over medium heat. Once hot, cook the garlic and ginger for about minute or until aromatic.

2. Turn the heat to a simmer and add in the lemon, turmeric, coconut milk, soy sauce, coconut sugar,

salt and nutmeg; continue to simmer for 1 minute or until heated through.

3.   Bon appétit!

Nutrition Info: Per Serving: Calories: 68; Fat: 5.1g; Carbs: 4.7g; Protein: 1.4g

Peanut Butter Shake

Servings: 2

Cooking Time: 5 Minutes

Ingredients:

- 1 cup plant-based milk
- 1 handful kale
- 2 bananas, frozen
- 2 Tbsp peanut butter
- ½ tsp ground cinnamon
- ¼ tsp vanilla powder

Directions:

1. Use a blender to combine all the ingredients for your shake.
2. Enjoy it!

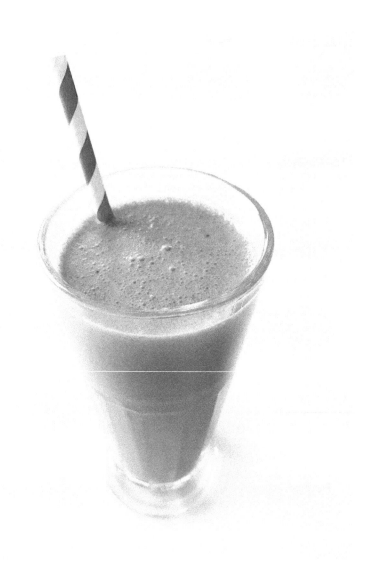

Hibiscus Tea

Servings: 2

Cooking Time: 5 Minutes

Ingredients:

- 1 tablespoon of raisins, diced
- 6 Almonds, raw and unsalted
- ½ teaspoon of hibiscus powder
- 2 cups of water

Directions:

1. Bring the water to a boil in a small saucepan, add in the hibiscus powder and raisins. Give it a good stir, cover and let simmer for a further two minutes.

2. Strain into a teapot and serve with a side helping of almonds.

3. Tips:

4. As an alternative to this tea, do not strain it and serve with the raisin pieces still swirling around in the teacup.

5. You could also serve this tea chilled for those hotter days.

6. Double or triple the recipe to provide you with iced-tea to enjoy during the week without having to make a fresh pot each time.

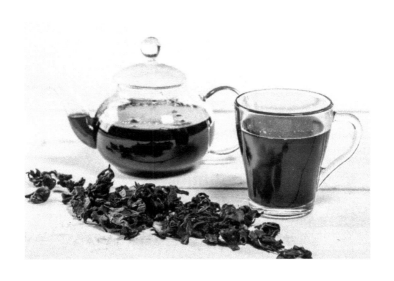

Barbecue Tahini Sauce

Servings: 8

Cooking Time: 0 Minute

Ingredients:

- 6 tablespoons tahini
- 3/4 teaspoon garlic powder
- 1/8 teaspoon red chili powder
- 2 teaspoons maple syrup
- 1/4 teaspoon salt
- 3 teaspoons molasses
- 3 teaspoons apple cider vinegar
- 1/4 teaspoon liquid smoke
- 10 teaspoons tomato paste
- 1/2 cup water

Directions:

1. Place all the ingredients in the order in a food processor or blender and then pulse for 3 to 5 minutes at high speed until smooth.
2. Tip the sauce in a bowl and then serve.

Nutrition Info: Calories: 86 Cal; Fat: 5 g: Carbs: 7 g;

rotein: 2 g; Fiber: 0 g

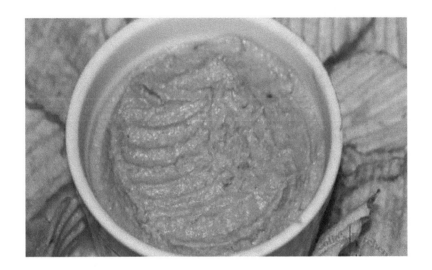

Strawberry Grapefruit Smoothie

Servings: 2

Cooking Time: 5 Minutes

Ingredients:

- 1 banana
- ½ cup strawberries, frozen
- 1 grapefruit
- ¼ cup milk
- ¼ cup plain yoghurt
- 2 Tbsp honey
- ½ tsp ginger, chopped

Directions:

1. Using a mixer, blend all the ingredients.
2. When smooth, top your drink with a slice of grapefruit and enjoy it!

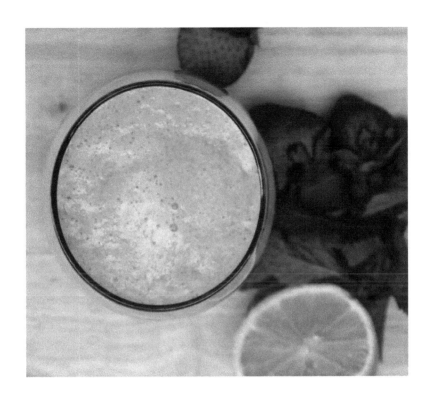

Easiest Vegan Mayo Ever

Servings: 6

Cooking Time: 15 Minutes

Ingredients:

- 1/2 cup olive oil, at room temperature
- 1/4 cup rice milk, unsweetened, at room temperature
- 1 teaspoon yellow mustard
- 1 tablespoon fresh lemon juice
- 1/3 teaspoon kosher salt

Directions:

1. Blend the milk, mustard, lemon juice and salt using your high-speed blender.

2. While the machine is going, gradually add in the olive oil and continue to blend at a low speed until the mixture has thickened.

3. Store in your refrigerator for about 6 days. Bon appétit!

Nutrition Info: Per Serving: Calories: 167; Fat: 18.1g; Carbs: 0.7g; Protein: 0.4g

Vegan Buffalo Sauce

Servings: 1

Cooking Time: 5 Minutes

Ingredients:

- 1/2 cup soy milk
- 1 cup hot sauce
- 1/2 cup vinegar
- 1/2 teaspoon pepper
- 2 tablespoons sugar
- 1/2 teaspoon garlic granules
- 1 tablespoon tomato sauce

Directions:

1. Mix soy milk, hot sauce, sugar, vinegar, sugar, pepper, tomato sauce and garlic granules in a pan and cook over medium heat for minutes.

2. Let cool and serve.

Vodka Cream Sauce

Servings: 1

Cooking Time: 5 Minutes

Ingredients:

- 1/4 cup cashews, unsalted, soaked in warm water for 15 minutes
- 24-ounce marinara sauce
- 2 tablespoons vodka
- 1/4 cup water

Directions:

1. Drain the cashews, transfer them in a food processor, pour in water, and blend for 2 minutes until smooth.

2. Tip the mixture in a pot, stir in pasta sauce and vodka and simmer for 3 minutes over medium heat until done, stirring constantly.

3. Serve sauce over pasta.

Nutrition Info: Calories: 207 Cal; Fat: 16 g: Carbs: 9.2 g; Protein: 2.4 g; Fiber: 4.3 g

Cilantro And Parsley Hot Sauce

Servings: 4

Cooking Time: 0 Minute

Ingredients:

*   2 cups of parsley and cilantro leaves with stems
*   4 Thai bird chilies, destemmed, deseeded, torn
*   2 teaspoons minced garlic
*   1 teaspoon salt
*   1/4 teaspoon coriander seed, ground
*   1/4 teaspoon ground black pepper
*   1/2 teaspoon cumin seeds, ground
*   3 green cardamom pods, toasted, ground
*   1/2 cup olive oil

Directions:

1. Take a spice blender or a food processor, place all the ingredients in it, and process for 5 minutes until the smooth paste comes together.
2. Serve straight away.

Nutrition Info: Calories: 130 Cal; Fat: 14 g: Carbs: 2 g; Protein: 1 g; Fiber: 1 g

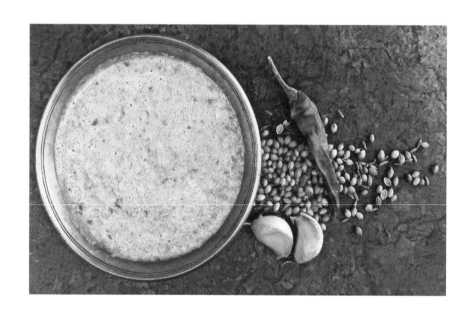

Incredible Barbecue Sauce

Servings: 68

Cooking Time: 6 Hours

Ingredients:

- 1/2 cup of chopped white onion
- 1 tablespoon of salt
- 1/4 cup of brown sugar
- 1/2 teaspoon of ground black pepper
- 4 teaspoons of paprika
- 2 tablespoons of molasses
- 1 tablespoon of apple cider vinegar
- 2 tablespoons of Worcestershire sauce
- 1 tablespoon of ground whole-grain mustard paste
- 4 cups of tomato ketchup
- 1/2 cup of water

Directions:

1. Using a 6-quarts slow cooker, place all the ingredients except for the salt, cilantro, and stir properly 2. Cover it with the lid, plug in the slow cooker and let it cook for 6 hours on the low heat setting or until it is cooked thoroughly.

3.   When the cooking time is over, with an immersion blender, process the sauce.

4.   Then continue cooking for 2 hours. While still stirring occasionally.

5.   Let the sauce cool off completely and serve or store in sterilized jars.

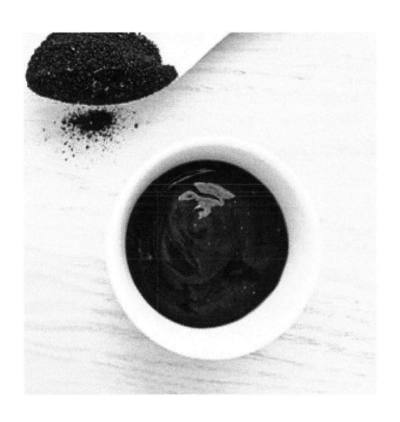

Ginger Smoothie with Citrus and Mint

Servings: 3

Cooking Time: 3 Minutes

Ingredients:

- 1 head Romaine lettuce, chopped into 4 chunks
- 2 Tbsp hemp seeds
- 5 mandarin oranges, peeled
- 1 banana, frozen
- 1 carrot
- 2-3 mint leaves
- ½ piece ginger root, peeled
- 1 cup water
- ¼ lemon, peeled
- ½ cup ice

Directions:

1. Put all the smoothie ingredients in a blender and blend until smooth.
2. Enjoy!

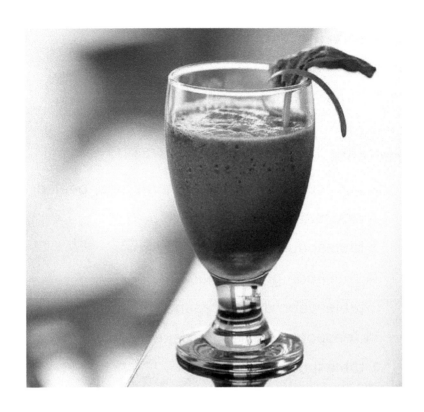

Spicy Red Wine Tomato Sauce

Servings: 4

Cooking Time: 1 Hour

Ingredients:

* 28 ounces puree of whole tomatoes, peeled
* 4 cloves of garlic, peeled
* 1 tablespoon dried basil
* ¼ teaspoon ground black pepper
* 1 tablespoon dried oregano
* ¼ teaspoon red pepper flakes
* 1 tablespoon dried sage
* 1 tablespoon dried thyme
* 3 teaspoon coconut sugar
* 1/2 of lemon, juice
* 1/4 cup red wine

Directions:

1. Take a large saucepan, place it over medium heat, add tomatoes and remaining ingredients, stir and simmer for hour or more until thickened and cooked.

2. Serve sauce over pasta.

Nutrition Info: Calories: 110 Cal; Fat: 2.5 g: Carbs: 9 g; Protein: 2 g; Fiber: 2 g

Green Goddess Hummus

Servings: 6

Cooking Time: 0 Minute

Ingredients:

- ¼ cup tahini
- ¼ cup lemon juice
- 2 tablespoons olive oil
- ½ cup chopped parsley
- ¼ cup chopped basil
- 3 tablespoons chopped chives
- 1 large clove of garlic, peeled, chopped
- ½ teaspoon salt
- 15-ounce cooked chickpeas
- 2 tablespoons water

Directions:

1. Place all the ingredients in the order in a food processor or blender and then pulse for 3 to 5 minutes at high speed until the thick mixture comes together.
2. Tip the hummus in a bowl and then serve.

Nutrition Info: Calories: 110.4 Cal; Fat: 6 g: Carbs: 1.5 g; Protein: 4.8 g; Fiber: 2.6 g

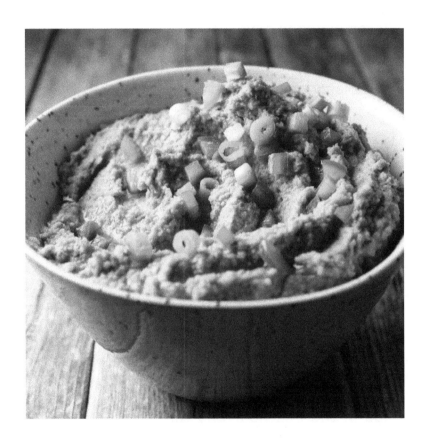

Classic Alfredo Sauce

Servings: 4

Cooking Time: 10 Minutes

Ingredients:

- 2 tablespoons olive oil
- 2 cloves garlic, minced
- 2 tablespoons rice flour
- 1 ½ cups rice milk, unsweetened
- Sea salt and ground black pepper, to taste
- 1/2 teaspoon red pepper flakes, crushed
- 4 tablespoons tahini
- 2 tablespoons nutritional yeast

Directions:

1. In a large saucepan, heat the olive oil over a moderate heat. Once hot, sauté the garlic for about 30 seconds or until fragrant.

2. Add in the rice flour and turn the heat to a simmer. Gradually add in the milk and continue to cook for a few minutes more, whisking constantly to avoid the lumps.

3. Add in the salt, black pepper, red pepper flakes, tahini and nutritional yeast.

.   Continue to cook on low until the sauce has thickened.

.   Store in an airtight container in your refrigerator for up to four days. Bon appétit!

Nutrition Info: Per Serving: Calories: 245; Fat: 17.9g;

Carbs: 14.9g; Protein: 8.2g

Authentic French Remoulade

Servings: 9

Cooking Time: 10 Minutes

Ingredients:

- 1 cup vegan mayonnaise
- 1 tablespoon Dijon mustard
- 1 scallion, finely chopped
- 1 teaspoon garlic, minced
- 2 tablespoons capers, coarsely chopped
- 1 tablespoon hot sauce
- 1 tablespoon fresh lemon juice
- 1 tablespoon flat-leaf parsley, chopped

Directions:

1. Thoroughly combine all the ingredients in your food processor or blender.
2. Blend until uniform and creamy.
3. Bon appétit!

Nutrition Info: Per Serving: Calories: 121; Fat: 10.4g; Carbs: 1.3g; Protein: 6.2g

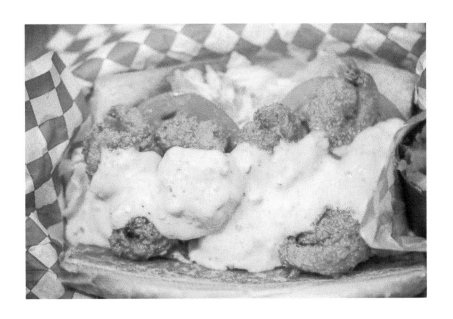

Energizing Ginger Detox Tonic

Servings: 2

Cooking Time: 10 Minutes

Ingredients:

- 1/2 teaspoon of grated ginger, fresh
- 1 small lemon slice
- 1/8 teaspoon of cayenne pepper
- 1/8 teaspoon of ground turmeric
- 1/8 teaspoon of ground cinnamon
- 1 teaspoon of maple syrup
- 1 teaspoon of apple cider vinegar
- 2 cups of boiling water

Directions:

1. Pour the boiling water into a small saucepan, add and stir the ginger, then let it rest for 8 to minutes, before covering the pan.

2. Pass the mixture through a strainer and into the liquid, add the cayenne pepper, turmeric, cinnamon and stir properly.

3. Add the maple syrup, vinegar, and lemon slice.

4. Add and stir an infused lemon and serve immediately.

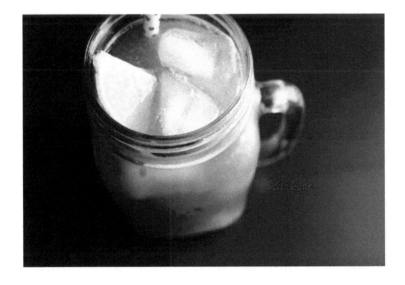

Marinara Sauce

Servings: 8

Cooking Time: 22 Minutes

Ingredients:

* 1/3 cup olive oil
* 1 can tomato paste
* 2 cans stewed tomatoes
* ½ cup white wine
* ¼ cup fresh parsley, chopped
* 1 teaspoon dried oregano, crushed
* Salt and ground black pepper, as required
* 1/3 cup olive oil
* 1/3 cup onion, chopped finely
* 1 garlic clove, minced

Directions:

1. Add the tomato paste, stewed tomatoes, garlic, parsley and oregano to a blender and blend until smooth.
2. Heat oil over medium heat and sauté chopped onions for minutes.

. Add the tomato mixture and wine and cook for about 20 minutes, stirring constantly.

. Remove from the flame and serve when cool.

Lemon And Rosemary Iced Tea

Servings: 4

Cooking Time: 10 Minutes

Ingredients:

* 4 cups of water
* 4 earl grey tea bags
* ¼ cup of sugar
* 2 lemons
* 1 sprig of rosemary

Directions:

1. Peel the two lemons and set the fruit aside.

2. In a medium saucepan, over medium heat combine the water, sugar, and lemon peels. Bring this to a boil.

3. Remove from the heat and place the rosemary and tea into the mixture. Cover the saucepan and steep for five minutes.

4. Add the juice of the two peeled lemons to the mixture, strain, chill, and serve.

5. Tips: Skip the sugar and use honey to taste.

5.   Do not squeeze the tea bags as they can cause the tea to become bitter.

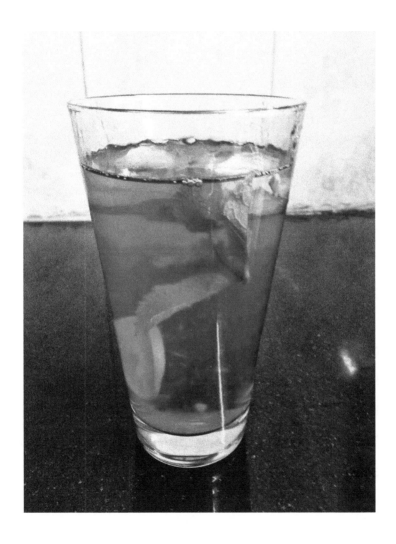

Almond And Sunflower Seed Mayo

Servings: 12

Cooking Time: 10 Minutes

Ingredients:

- 1/4 cup raw sunflower seeds, hulled
- 1/2 cup raw almonds
- 3/4 cup water
- 1/2 teaspoon onion powder
- 1/2 teaspoon garlic powder
- 1/4 teaspoon dried dill
- 1/2 teaspoon sea salt
- 1 cup sunflower seed oil
- 2 tablespoons fresh lime juice
- 1 tablespoon apple cider vinegar

Directions:

1. Process all the ingredients, except for the oil, in your blender or food processor until well combined.
2. Then, gradually add in the oil and continue to blend at low speed until smooth and creamy.
3. Add more spices, if needed.

4. Place in your refrigerator until ready to serve. Bon
   appétit!

Nutrition Info: Per Serving: Calories: 109; Fat: 9.2g;
Carbs: 4.4g; Protein: 3.7g

Classic Homemade Ketchup

Servings: 10

Cooking Time: 25 Minutes

Ingredients:

- 4 ounces canned tomato paste
- 2 tablespoons agave syrup
- 1/4 cup red wine vinegar
- 1/4 cup water
- 1/2 teaspoon kosher salt
- 1/4 teaspoon garlic powder

Directions:

1.   Preheat a saucepan over medium flame. Then, add all the ingredients to a saucepan and bring it to a boil.

2.   Turn the heat to a simmer; let it simmer, stirring continuously, for about minutes or until the sauce has thickened.

3.   Store in a glass jar in your refrigerator. Bon appétit!

Nutrition Info: Per Serving: Calories: 24; Fat: 0g; Carbs: 5.5g; Protein: 0.5g

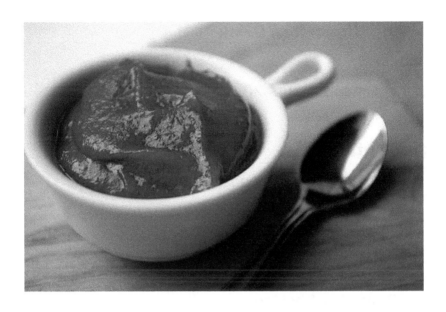

Soothing Ginger Tea Drink

Servings: 8

Cooking Time: 2 Hours 20 Minutes

Ingredients:

- 1 tablespoon of minced gingerroot
- 2 tablespoons of honey
- 15 green tea bags
- 32 fluid ounce of white grape juice
- 2 quarts of boiling water

Directions:

1. Pour water into a 4-quarts slow cooker, immerse tea bags, cover the cooker and let stand for minutes. 2. After 10 minutes, remove and discard tea bags and stir in remaining ingredients.

3. Return cover to slow cooker, then plug in and let cook at high heat setting for 2 hours or until heated through.

4. When done, strain the liquid and serve hot or cold.

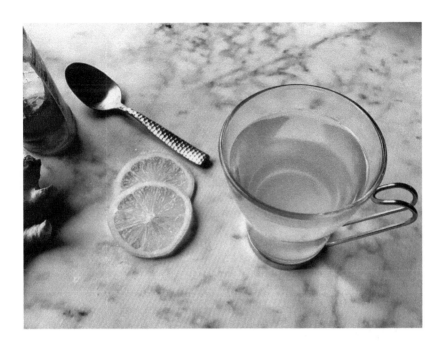

Herb Avocado Salad Dressing

Servings: 6

Cooking Time: 10 Minutes

Ingredients:

- 1 medium-sized avocado, pitted, peeled and mashed
- 4 tablespoons extra-virgin olive oil
- 4 tablespoons almond milk
- 2 tablespoons cilantro, minced
- 2 tablespoons parsley, minced
- 1 lemon, juiced
- 2 garlic cloves, minced
- 1/2 teaspoon mustard seeds
- 1/2 teaspoon red pepper flakes
- Kosher salt and cayenne pepper, to taste

Directions:

1. Mix all the above ingredients in your food processor or blender.
2. Blend until uniform, smooth and creamy.
3. Bon appétit!

Nutrition Info: Per Serving: Calories: 101; Fat: 9.4g; Carbs: 4.3g; Protein: 1.2g

Brownie Batter Orange Chia Shake

Servings: 2

Cooking Time: 0 Minute

Ingredients:

- 2 tablespoons cocoa powder
- 3 tablespoons chia seeds
- ¼ teaspoon salt
- 4 tablespoons chocolate chips
- 4 teaspoons coconut sugar
- ½ teaspoon orange zest
- ½ teaspoon vanilla extract, unsweetened
- 2 cup almond milk

Directions:

1.   Place all the ingredients in the order in a food processor or blender and then pulse for 2 to 3 minutes at high speed until smooth.

2.   Pour the smoothie into two glasses and then serve.

Vegan Ranch Dressing

Servings: 16

Cooking Time: 0 Minute

Ingredients:

- 1/4 teaspoon. ground black pepper
- 2 teaspoon. chopped parsley
- 1/2 teaspoon. garlic powder • 1 tablespoon chopped dill
- 1/2 teaspoon. onion powder
- 1 cup vegan mayonnaise
- 1/2 cup soy milk, unsweetened

Directions:

1. Take a medium bowl, add all the ingredients in it and then whisk until combined.
2. Serve straight away

Nutrition Info: Calories: 16 Cal ;Fat: 9 g :Carbs: 0 g ;Protein: 0 g ;Fiber: 0 g

Barbecue Sauce

Servings: 16

Cooking Time: 0 Minute

Ingredients:

8 ounces tomato sauce

1 teaspoon garlic powder

¼ teaspoon ground black pepper

1/2 teaspoon. sea salt

2 Tablespoons Dijon mustard

3 packets stevia

1 teaspoon molasses

1 Tablespoon apple cider vinegar

2 Tablespoons tamari

1 teaspoon liquid aminos

Directions:

.   Take a medium bowl, place all the ingredients in it, and stir until combined.

2.   Serve straight away

Nutrition Info: Calories: 29 Cal; Fat: 0.1 g: Carbs: 7 g; Protein: 0.1 g; Fiber: 0.1 g

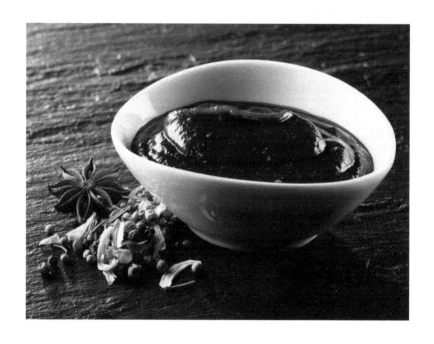

Strawberry Pink Drink

Servings: 4

Cooking Time: 5 Minutes

Ingredients:

- Water (1 C., Boiling)
- Sugar (2 T.)
- Acai Tea Bag (1)
- Coconut Milk (1 C.)
- Frozen Strawberries (1/2 C.)

Directions:

1. If you are looking for a little treat, this is going to be the recipe for you! You will begin by boiling your cup of water and seep the tea bag in for at least five minutes.

2. When the tea is set, add in the sugar and coconut milk. Be sure to stir well to spread the sweetness throughout the tea.

3. Finally, add in your strawberries, and you can enjoy your freshly made pink drink!

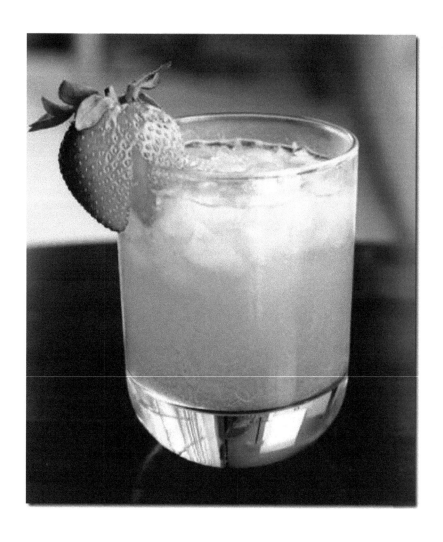

Simple Almond Butter Fudge

Servings: 8

Cooking Time: 0 Minutes

Ingredients:

- 1/2 cup almond butter
- 15 drops liquid stevia
- 2 1/2 tbsp coconut oil

Directions:

1. Combine together almond butter and coconut oil in a saucepan. Gently warm until melted.

2. Add stevia and stir well.

3. Pour mixture into the candy container and place in refrigerator until set.

4. Serve and enjoy.

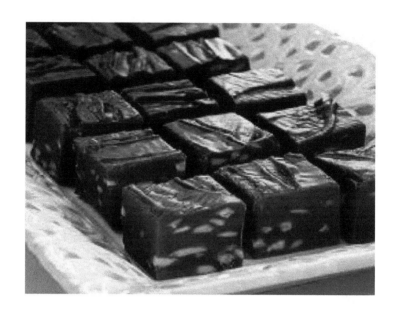

General Tso Sauce

Servings: 4

Cooking Time: 10 Minutes

Ingredients:

Rice Vinegar (1/4 C.)

Water (1/2 C.)

Sriracha Sauce (1 ½ T.)

Soy Sauce (1/4 C.)

Corn Starch (1 ½ T.)

Sugar (1/2 C.)

Directions:

1. General Tso Sauce is a classic, and you can now make a healthier version of it! All you have to do is take out your saucepan and place all of the ingredients in.

2. Once in place, bring everything over medium heat and whisk together for ten minutes or until the sauce begins to get thick.

3. Finally, remove from the heat and enjoy!

Rainbow Ketchup

Servings: 4

Cooking Time: 15 Minutes

Ingredients:

- ¾ teaspoon salt
- 1 cup strawberries, fresh
- 1 big bay leaf
- 1 teaspoon garlic, grated
- 1 cup onion, chopped
- ¼ cup apple cider vinegar
- 1/3 cup brown sugar

Directions:

1. Take a saucepan and add all the ingredients to it.
2. Cover it and cook for 15 minutes on medium heat
3. Uncover it and cook for another 15 minutes.
4. Remove from heat, store and enjoy.

Perfect Hollandaise Sauce

Servings: 6

Cooking Time: 15 Minutes

Ingredients:

- 1/2 cup cashews, soaked and drained
- 1 cup almond milk
- 2 tablespoons fresh lemon juice
- 3 tablespoons coconut oil
- 3 tablespoons nutritional yeast
- Sea salt and ground white pepper, to taste
- A pinch of grated nutmeg
- 1/2 teaspoon red pepper flakes, crushed

Directions:

1. Puree all the ingredients in a high-speed blender or food processor.

2. Then, heat the mixture in a small saucepan over low-medium heat; cook, stirring occasionally, until the sauce has reduced and thickened.

3. Bon appétit!

Nutrition Info: Per Serving: Calories: 145; Fat: 12.6g;

Carbs: 6.1g; Protein: 3.3g

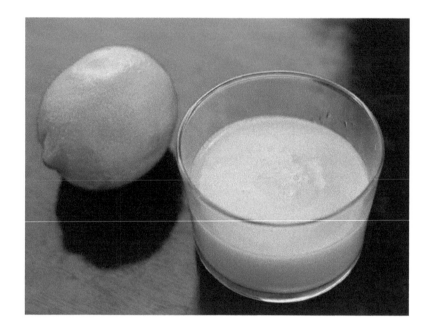

Avocado Pudding

Servings: 8

Cooking Time: 0 Minute

Ingredients:

- 2 ripe avocados, peeled, pitted and cut into pieces
- 1 tbsp fresh lime juice
- 14 oz can coconut milk
- 80 drops of liquid stevia
- 2 tsp vanilla extract

Directions:

1. Add all ingredients into the blender and blend until smooth.
2. Serve and enjoy.

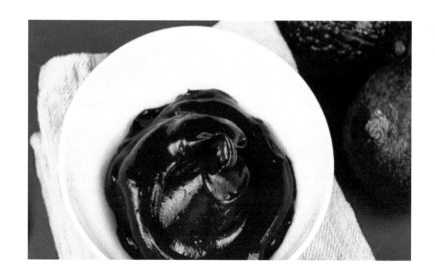

Creamy Mustard Sauce

Servings: 4

Cooking Time: 35 Minutes

Ingredients:

1/2 plain hummus

1 teaspoon fresh garlic, minced

1 tablespoon deli mustard

1 tablespoon extra-virgin olive oil

1 tablespoon fresh lime juice

1 teaspoon red pepper flakes

1/2 teaspoon sea salt

1/4 teaspoon ground black pepper

Directions:

1. Thoroughly combine all ingredients in a mixing bowl.

2. Let it sit in your refrigerator for about 30 minutes before serving.

3. Bon appétit!

Nutrition Info: Per Serving: Calories: 73; Fat: 4.2g; Carbs: 7.1g; Protein: 1.7g

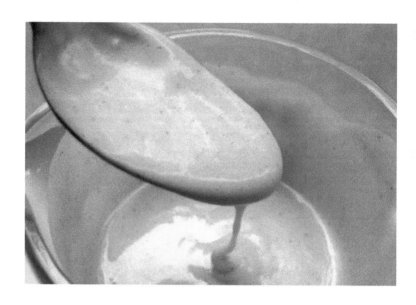

Tangy Tomato Sauce

Servings: 50

Cooking Time: 12 Hours

Ingredients:

- 10 tomatoes, peeled and seeded
- Half of a small white onion, peeled and chopped
- 1 teaspoon of minced garlic
- 1 teaspoon of salt
- 1 teaspoon of ground black pepper
- 1 teaspoon of ground cayenne pepper
- 1 teaspoon of dried oregano
- 1 teaspoon of dried basil
- 1/8 teaspoon of ground cinnamon
- 1/4 cup of olive oil

Directions:

1. Crush the tomatoes and add it to a 6-quarts slow cooker along with the remaining ingredients.

2. Stir properly and cover it with the lid.

3. Plug in the slow cooker and let it cook for 12 hours at the low heat setting or until it is cooked thoroughly, while still stirring occasionally.

4.   Let the sauce cool off completely and serve or store in sterilized jars.

Runner Recovery Bites

Servings: 12

Cooking Time: 10 Minutes

Ingredients:

1/4 cup pumpkin seeds, soaked for 1 hour

1/3 cup oats

1/4 cup sunflower seeds, soaked for 1 hour

5 dates

1 teaspoon maca powder

1 tablespoon goji berries

1 teaspoon coconut, shredded and unsweetened

1 tablespoon coconut water

1 teaspoon vanilla extract

1 tablespoon protein powder

1 tablespoon maple syrup

1/4 cup hemp seeds

A pinch sea salt

Directions:

1. Drain sunflower and pumpkin seeds and add to a blender. Blend until a paste forms. Add dates and

blend to mix. Add the remaining ingredients except hemp seeds and blend until a dough forms.

2. Roll 1 tablespoon dough into balls with hands. Roll the ball in hemp seeds until covered.

3. Transfer the prepared balls to a plate and freeze until firm.

4. Serve and enjoy.

Warm Spiced Lemon Drink

Servings: 12

Cooking Time: 2 Hours

Ingredients:

1 cinnamon stick, about 3 inches long

1/2 teaspoon of whole cloves

2 cups of coconut sugar

4 fluid of ounce pineapple juice

1/2 cup and 2 tablespoons of lemon juice

12 fluid ounce of orange juice

2 1/2 quarts of water

Directions:

. Pour water into a 6-quarts slow cooker and stir the sugar and lemon juice properly.

. Wrap the cinnamon, the whole cloves in cheesecloth and tie its corners with string.

. Immerse this cheesecloth bag in the liquid present in the slow cooker and cover it with the lid.

. Then plug in the slow cooker and let it cook on high heat setting for 2 hours or until it is heated thoroughly.

5.   When done, discard the cheesecloth bag and serve the drink hot or cold.

Fragrant Spiced Coffee

Servings: 8

Cooking Time: 3 Hours

Ingredients:

- 4 cinnamon sticks, each about 3 inches long
- 1 1/2 teaspoons of whole cloves
- 1/3 cup of honey
- 2-ounce of chocolate syrup
- 1/2 teaspoon of anise extract
- 8 cups of brewed coffee

Directions:

1.   Pour the coffee in a 4-quarts slow cooker and pour in the remaining ingredients except for cinnamon and stir properly.

2.   Wrap the whole cloves in cheesecloth and tie its corners with strings.

3.   Immerse this cheesecloth bag in the liquid present in the slow cooker and cover it with the lid.

4.   Then plug in the slow cooker and let it cook on the low heat setting for 3 hours or until heated thoroughly. 5. When done, discard the cheesecloth bag and serve.

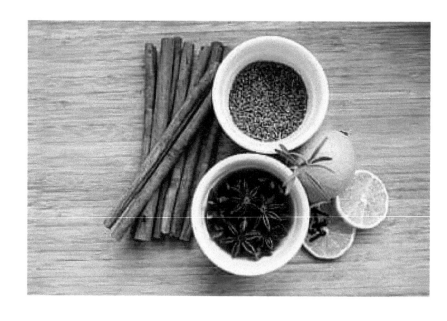

Nacho Cheese Sauce

Servings: 12

Cooking Time: 5 Minutes

Ingredients:

2 cups cashews, unsalted, soaked in warm water for 15 minutes

2 teaspoons salt

1/2 cup nutritional yeast

1 teaspoon garlic powder

1/2 teaspoon smoked paprika

1/2 teaspoon red chili powder

1 teaspoon onion powder

2 teaspoons Sriracha

3 tablespoons lemon juice

4 cups water, divided

Directions:

1. Drain the cashews, transfer them to a food processor, then add remaining ingredients, reserving 3 cups water, and, and pulse for 3 minutes until smooth. 2. Tip the mixture in a saucepan, place it over medium heat and

cook for 3 to 5 minutes until the sauce has thickened and bubbling, whisking constantly.

3. When done, taste the sauce to adjust seasoning and then serve.

Nutrition Info: Calories: 128 Cal; Fat: 10 g: Carbs: 8 g; Protein: 5 g; Fiber: 1 g

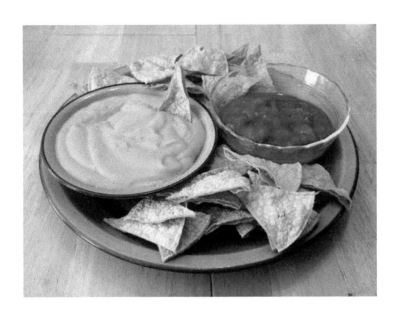

Berry Beet Velvet Smoothie

Servings: 1

Cooking Time: 0 Minute

Ingredients:

- 1/2 of frozen banana
- 1 cup mixed red berries
- 1 Medjool date, pitted
- 1 small beet, peeled, chopped
- 1 tablespoon cacao powder
- 1 teaspoon chia seeds
- 1/4 teaspoon vanilla extract, unsweetened
- 1/2 teaspoon lemon juice
- 2 teaspoons coconut butter
- 1 cup coconut milk, unsweetened

Directions:

1. Place all the ingredients in the order in a food processor or blender and then pulse for 2 to 3 minutes at high speed until smooth.

2. Pour the smoothie into a glass and then serve.

Nutrition Info: Calories: 234 Cal; Fat: 5 g: Carbs: 42 g; Protein: 11 g; Fiber: 7 g

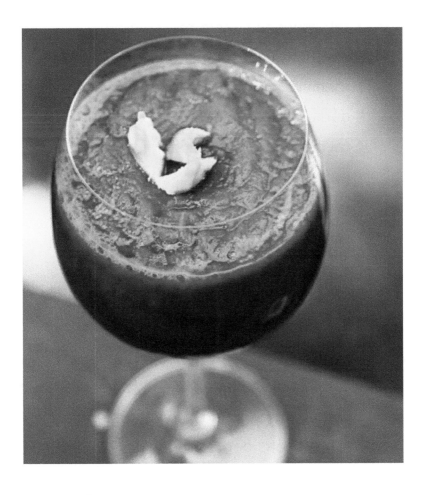

Spice Trade Beans and Bulgur

Servings: 10

Cooking Time: 2 Hours

Ingredients:

- 3 tablespoons canola oil, isolated
- 2 medium onions, slashed
- 1 medium sweet red pepper, slashed
- 5 garlic cloves, minced
- 1 tablespoon ground cumin
- 1 tablespoon paprika
- 2 teaspoons ground ginger
- 1 teaspoon pepper
- 1/2 teaspoon ground cinnamon
- 1/2 teaspoon cayenne pepper
- 1-1/2 cups bulgur
- 1 can (28 ounces) squashed tomatoes
- 1 can (14-1/2 ounces) diced tomatoes, undrained
- 1 container (32 ounces) vegetable juices
- 2 tablespoons darker sugar
- 2 tablespoons soy sauce
- 1 can (15 ounces) garbanzo beans or chickpeas, flushed and depleted

- 1/2 cup brilliant raisins
- Minced crisp cilantro, discretionary

Directions:

1. In a large skillet, heat 2 tablespoons oil over medium-high warmth. Include onions and pepper; cook and mix until delicate, 3-4 minutes. Include garlic and seasonings; cook brief longer. Move to a 5-qt. slow cooker.

2. In the same skillet, heat remaining oil over medium-high warmth. Include bulgur; cook and mix until daintily caramelized, 3 minutes or until softly sautéed.

3. Include bulgur, tomatoes, stock, darker sugar, and soy sauce to slow cooker. Cook, secured, on low 4 hours or until bulgur is delicate. Mix in beans and raisins; cook 30 minutes longer. Whenever wanted, sprinkle with cilantro.

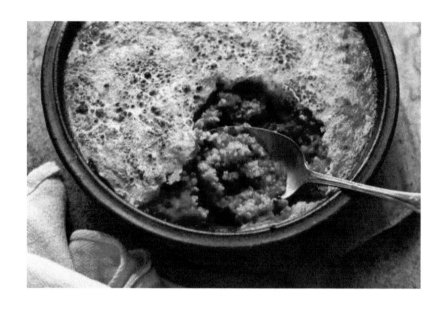

Classic Tofu Scramble

Servings: 2

Cooking Time: 15 Minutes

Ingredients:

1 tablespoon olive oil

6 ounces extra-firm tofu, pressed and crumbled

1 cup baby spinach

Sea salt and ground black pepper to taste

1/2 teaspoon turmeric powder

1/4 teaspoon cumin powder

1/2 teaspoon garlic powder

1 handful fresh chives, chopped

Directions:

1. Heat the olive oil in a frying skillet over medium heat. When it's hot, add the tofu and sauté for 8 minutes, stirring occasionally to promote even cooking.

2. Add in the baby spinach and aromatics and continue sautéing an additional 1 to minutes.

3. Garnish with fresh chives and serve warm. Bon appétit!

Nutrition Info: Per Serving: Calories: 202; Fat: 14.3g;

Carbs: 7.5g; Protein: 14.6g

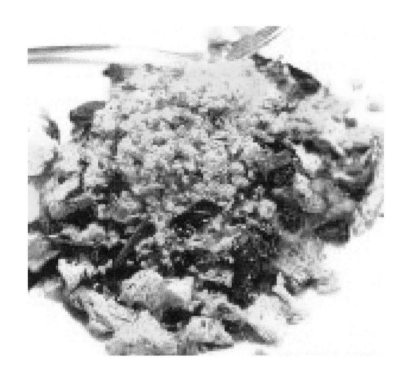

Almond & Raisin Granola

Servings: 8

Cooking Time: 20 Minutes

Ingredients:

- 5 ½ cups old-fashioned oats
- 1 ½ cups chopped walnuts
- ½ cup shelled sunflower seeds
- 1 cup golden raisins
- 1 cup shaved almonds
- 1 cup pure maple syrup
- ½ tsp ground cinnamon
- ¼ tsp ground allspice
- A pinch of salt

Directions:

1. Preheat oven to 325 F. In a baking dish, place the oats, walnuts and sunflower seeds. Bake for minutes. Lower the heat from the oven to 300 F. Stir in the raisins, almonds, maple syrup, cinnamon, allspice, and salt. Bake for an additional 15 minutes. Allow to cool before serving.

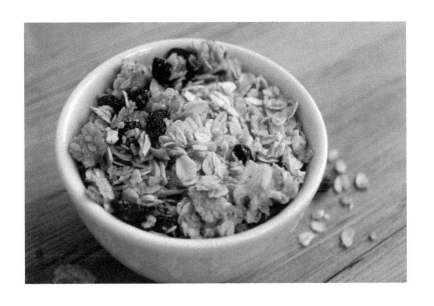

Pumpkin And Oatmeal Bars

Servings: 3

Cooking Time: 30 Minutes

Ingredients:

- 3 cups thick oatmeal
- 1 cup seedless dates
- ½ cup of boiling water
- 2 teaspoons pumpkin pie spice
- 1 tablespoon ground flaxseed or chia seeds
- ¼ cup small sliced nuts (optional)
- ¼ cup of vegetable milk
- 1 cup mashed pumpkin

Directions:

1. Preheat the oven to 350 degrees Fahrenheit.
2. Cut the date into small pieces, put them in a bowl, and pour hot water. Rest for 10 minutes.
3. Add dry ingredients to the bowl and mix well.
4. Add dates to the dry ingredients along with water, pumpkins, and plant milk and mix well.
5. Cover the square bread with baking paper and push the mixture firmly into the bread.

6.   Cook for 15-20 minutes.

7.   Allow the mixture to cool completely in the container, then cut into 16 squares or 8 large bars.

8.   Store in the refrigerator for up to 7 days.

Vegetarian Breakfast Casserole

Servings: 4

Cooking Time: 35 Minutes

Ingredients:

- 5 medium potatoes, about 22 ounces, boiled
- 10 ounces silken tofu
- 5 ounces tempeh, cubed
- 1 tablespoon chives, cut into rings
- 1 medium white onion, peeled chopped
- ¾ teaspoon ground black pepper
- 1 ½ teaspoon salt
- 1 teaspoon turmeric
- 2 1/2 teaspoons paprika powder
- 1 1/2 tablespoons olive oil
- 1 tablespoon corn starch
- 1 teaspoon soy sauce
- 1 tablespoon barbecue sauce
- 1/2 teaspoon liquid smoke
- 1/2 cup vegan cheese

Directions:

1. Switch on the oven, then set it to 350 degrees F and let it preheat.

2. Meanwhile, peel the boiled potatoes, then cut them into cubes and set aside until required.

3. Prepare tempeh and for this, take a skillet pan, place it over medium heat, add half of the oil, and when hot, add half of the onion and cook for 1 minute.

4. Then add tempeh pieces, season with 1 teaspoon paprika, add soy sauce, liquid smoke and BBQ sauce, season with salt and black pepper and cook tempeh for 5 minutes, set aside until required.

5. Take a large skillet pan, place it over medium heat, add remaining oil and onion and cook for 2 minutes until beginning to soften.

6. Then add potatoes, season with ½ teaspoon paprika, salt, and black pepper to taste and cook for 5 minutes until crispy, set aside until required.

7. Take a medium bowl, place tofu in it, then add remaining ingredients and whisk until smooth.

8. Take a casserole dish, place potatoes and tempeh in it, top with tofu mixture, sprinkle some more cheese, and bake for 20 minutes until done.

9.   Serve straight away.

Nutrition Info: Calories: 212 Cal; Fat: 7 g: Carbs: 28 g; Protein: 11 g; Fiber: 5 g

Vegan Banh Mi

Servings: 4

Cooking Time: 35 Minutes

Ingredients:

1/2 cup rice vinegar

1/4 cup water

1/4 cup white sugar

2 carrots, cut into 1/16-inch-thick matchsticks • 1/2 cup white (daikon radish, cut into 1/16-inchthick matchsticks

1 white onion, thinly sliced

2 tablespoons olive oil

12 ounces firm tofu, cut into sticks

1/4 cup vegan mayonnaise

1 ½ tablespoons soy sauce

2 cloves garlic, minced

1/4 cup fresh parsley, chopped

Kosher salt and ground black pepper, to taste

2 standard French baguettes, cut into four pieces

4 tablespoons fresh cilantro, chopped

4 lime wedges

Directions:

1. Bring the rice vinegar, water and sugar to a boil and stir until the sugar has dissolved, about minute. Allow it to cool.

2. Pour the cooled vinegar mixture over the carrot, daikon radish and onion; allow the vegetables to marinate for at least 30 minutes.

3. While the vegetables are marinating, heat the olive oil in a frying pan over medium-high heat. Once hot, add the tofu and sauté for 8 minutes, stirring occasionally to promote even cooking.

4. Then, mix the mayo, soy sauce, garlic, parsley, salt and ground black pepper in a small bowl.

5. Slice each piece of the baguette in half the long way. Then, toast the baguette halves under the preheated broiler for about 3 minutes.

6. To assemble the banh mi sandwiches, spread each half of the toasted baguette with the mayonnaise mixture; fill the cavity of the bottom half of the bread with the fried tofu sticks, marinated vegetables and cilantro leaves.

7. Lastly, squeeze the lime wedges over the filling and top with the other half of the baguette. Bon appétit!

Nutrition Info: Per Serving: Calories: 372; Fat: 21.9g; Carbs: 29.5g; Protein: 17.6g

Blueberry Smoothie Bowl

Servings: 2

Cooking Time: 5 Minutes

Ingredients:

- 1 tbsp. ground flaxseed
- 1 medium banana
- 4 ice cubes
- 1 cup blueberries
- ¾ cup unsweetened almond milk
- 1 tbsp. maple syrup
- ¼ cup nuts chopped

Directions:

1. Blend all ingredients in high speed blender.
2. The mixture will be rather thick so make sure you have a good high-speed blender.
3. If you prefer a thinner consistency add more almond milk.
4. Garnish with chopped nuts and mint leaves.
5. Serve and enjoy!

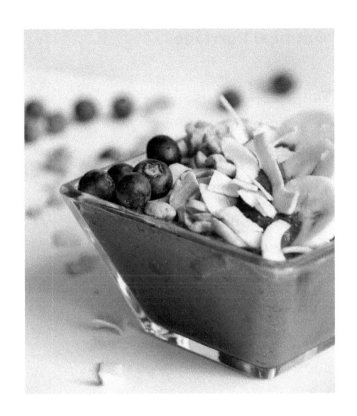

Almond Oatmeal Porridge

Servings: 4

Cooking Time: 25 Minutes

Ingredients:

- 2 ½ cups vegetable broth
- 2 ½ cups almond milk
- ½ cup steel-cut oats
- 1 tbsp pearl barley
- ½ cup slivered almonds
- ¼ cup nutritional yeast
- 2 cups old-fashioned rolled oats

Directions:

1. Pour the broth and almond milk in a pot over medium heat and bring to a boil. Stir in oats, pearl barley, almond slivers, and nutritional yeast. Reduce the heat and simmer for 20 minutes. Add in the rolled oats, cook for an additional 5 minutes, until creamy. Allow to cool before serving.

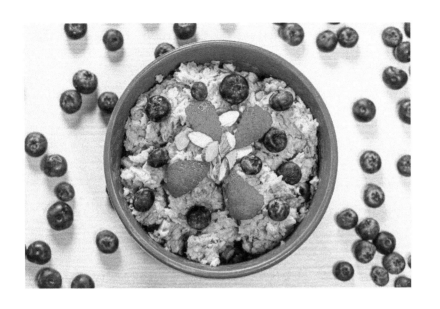

The Quick and Easy Bowl of Oatmeal for Breakfast

Servings: 2

Cooking Time: 5 Minutes

Ingredients:

- ½ cup of quick oatmeal
- ½ - ⅔ cup of hot or cold water
- ½ cup of vegetable milk
- 1 teaspoon of maqui berry powder or acai powder (optional)
- ½ cup of fresh grapes or berries
- banana (or a whole banana, if you prefer)
- Walnuts
- Seeds

Directions:

1. Combine oatmeal and water in a bowl, and let them soak for a few minutes.
2. Cut the banana and grapes or berries as you wish, and add them to the oatmeal.
3. Pour vegetable milk over oatmeal and fruits.
4. Cover with nuts, seeds, powdered maqui berry or acai powder. I use walnuts and hemp seeds.

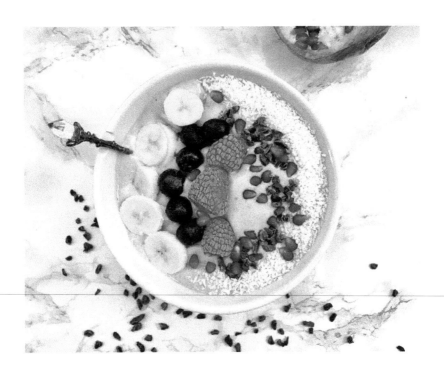

Orange French Toast

Servings: 4

Cooking Time: 10 Minutes

Ingredients:

- 3 very ripe bananas
- 1 cup unsweetened nondairy milk
- zest and juice of 1 orange
- 1 teaspoon ground cinnamon
- ¼ teaspoon grated nutmeg
- 4 slices french bread
- 1 tablespoon coconut oil

Directions:

1. Preparing the Ingredients.

2. In a blender, combine the bananas, almond milk, orange juice and zest, cinnamon, and nutmeg, then blend until smooth. Pour the mixture into a 9-by-13-inch baking dish. Soak the bread in the mixture for 5 minutes on each side.

3. Cook

4. While the bread soaks, heat a griddle or sauté pan over medium-high heat. Melt the coconut oil in the

pan and swirl to coat. Cook the bread slices until golden brown on both sides for about 5 minutes each. Serve immediately.

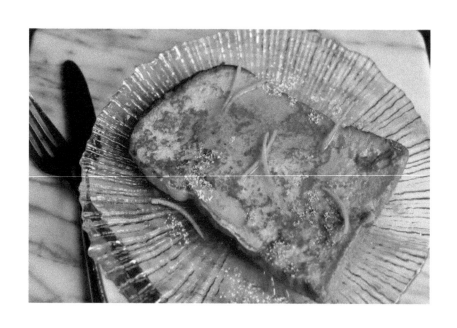

Lightning Source UK Ltd.
Milton Keynes UK
UKHW020810080621
385129UK00001B/86

9 781803 171562